THE BASICS OF
DIABETES NUTRITIONAL THERAPY
FOR AFRICAN AMERICANS

THE BASICS OF
DIABETES NUTRITIONAL THERAPY
FOR AFRICAN AMERICANS

A PRIMER FOR DIABETES MEAL PLANNING
IN THE PRIMARY CARE SETTING

Cheryl Campbell Atkinson
PhD, RD, LDN

iUniverse, Inc.
New York Lincoln Shanghai

THE BASICS OF
DIABETES NUTRITIONAL THERAPY
FOR AFRICAN AMERICANS
A Primer For Diabetes Meal Planning
In The Primary Care Setting

iUniverse, Inc.

For information address:
iUniverse, Inc.
2021 Pine Lake Road, Suite 100
Lincoln, NE 68512
www.iuniverse.com

*These basic guidelines have been prepared primarily
for use by
non-nutrition health care professionals.*

This manual is intended for informational purposes only and is not to be
used in place of appropriate medical care. Health care professionals who use
this manual are advised to consult with a licensed physician and or a
registered dietitian before making permanent changes in the medical
nutritional therapy of the clients in their care. With the availability of new
research finding, diabetes data is ever changing. The information in this
manual is the most current available.

ISBN: 0-595-32901-2

Printed in the United States of America

This book is dedicated to my father-in-law, Walsie Atkinson and my uncle, Burchell McGhie, who lived long and productive lives with type 2 diabetes. Their courage, spirit and zest for life were truly inspirations.

INTENDED USER

A PROFESSIONAL RESOURCE MANUAL

The basics of Diabetes nutritional therapy For African Americans; A primer for diabetes meal planning in the primary care setting is tailored to meet the varying educational backgrounds of most health care providers.

The medical nutrition therapy for diabetics is most appropriately designed and implemented by the skilled registered dietitian (RD). When an RD is not available, these responsibilities along with the subsequent monitoring of the patient will be the responsibility of a member of the health care team. This team member usually ends-up being a non-nutrition health professional. A diagnosis of diabetes can be devastating. This manual is designed to help the non-nutrition health professional obtain the basics necessary to provide initial counseling and/or monitoring of these patients, and in particular the African American patient with diabetes.

The diet (also called the meal plan), which is included as part of the Medical Nutrition Therapy (MNT) for diabetes, parallels that of a moderate heart healthy plan, and must be strongly encouraged. The control of diabetes works best when the meal plan is used in conjunction with the medical therapy, (which may include insulin and or medication), prescribed by the licensed physician.

This manual is a rich source of needed information for the non-nutrition health professional. This excellent counseling tool has been long needed in the public health primary care setting.
Stephanie Marshall MS, RD, LDN.

The integration of the cultural eating patterns, with the necessary medical nutrition therapy for diabetes will help patients more readily accept the life style modification necessary, with this chronic disease. This manual will be well utilized by health care professionals.
Lorna Shelton MS, RD, CDE.

CONTENTS

CHAPTER 1

INTRODUCTION

The United States is a melting pot of many cultures from around the world. This cultural diversity impacts what and how we eat. Presently, African Americans are the second largest minority group, and like many ethnic groups, they have been removed from their original homeland for several generations. Although African Americans now live in every state in the land, the lifestyle of parents and grandparents, who lived primarily in the southern United States, had the greatest influence on creating the social, religious and cultural traditions practiced by African Americans. These traditional practices, which have survived through today, have at their center, soul food cooking and feasting with family and friends.

The term 'soul-food' was coined to identify and describe the cooking practices used in the typical African American diet. Many of the foods used are rich in healthful nutrients, however the cooking methods and the combination of typical food items used increases the sodium, fat and sugar content of traditional dishes to extremely high levels.
African Americans have paid a high price for this lifestyle, with high incidences of diabetes.

Facts and Figures

Diabetes is the fourth leading cause of disease-related death for African Americans. When compared to Caucasians, African Americans are 1.7 times more likely to have diabetes. Data from the American Diabetes Association indicates that approximately 2.3 million or 10.8% of all African Americans have diabetes, and about one-third of them are unaware that they have this deadly disease. The prevalence of this disease is striking in this ethnic group. It affects all age groups, but seems to have a high prevalence with persons from the age of fifty-five years and older. Twenty five percent, or one-out-of-four, in this age group have diabetes.

1

What is Diabetes?

Diabetes is a disease that affects the body's ability to produce or respond to insulin. Insulin is the hormone that allows blood glucose (also called blood sugar) to enter the cells of the body to be used for energy. Diabetes causes blood glucose to buildup in the body adversely affecting several organs of the body (kidneys, eyes, heart,) and normal body processes, and may lead to death. This disease is chronic, and has no cure.

The complications that can be caused by diabetes are blindness, due to diabetic retinopathy; kidney disease due to diabetic nephropathy; heart disease and stroke; non-traumatic lower limb amputation; and impotence due to diabetic neuropathy or blood vessel blockage. Of these complications African Americans experience higher rates of blindness, kidney disease (failure), and amputation, than any other ethnic group.

CHAPTER 2

GENERAL GUIDELINES FOR BASIC DIABETES MEDICAL NUTRITION THERAPY

Healthy eating is one of the basic and important diabetes care tools. Controlling diabetes through nutrition therapy can improve long—term health and the quality of life.

The goals of nutrition self-management for Diabetes Mellitus are:

1. to maintain as near-normal blood glucose levels, by balancing food, insulin and exercise;
2. to prevent hyperglycemia and hypoglycemia and,
3. to reduce the risk of atherosclerosis and microvascular complications.

Almost all persons with diabetes can be considered to have non-insulin dependent (NIDDM) or insulin-dependent (IDDM). The specific dietary recommendations and any additional considerations will vary based on type of diabetes and the medical management program, of which the nutrition therapy plays a major part.

The target blood glucose control ranges in Diabetes are:

*   normal fasting plasma blood glucose: < 115 mg/dl
*   normal post prandial plasma blood glucose   < 140 mg/dl
*   normal glycosylate hemoglobin: HbAlc < 6 %

Non-insulin dependent diabetes mellitus and insulin dependent diabetes mellitus have distinctive features that are readily identifiable.

FEATURES OF IDDM AND NIDDM

	TYPE 1 (IDDM)	TYPE 2 (NIDDM)
Other names	Insulin dependent Juvenile-onset diabetes Ketosis-prone diabetes Brittle diabetes	Non-insulin dependent Adult-onset diabetes Ketosis-resistant diabetes Lipopiethoric diabetes Stable diabetes
Age of onset	<20 (mean age, 12)	>40
Associated conditions	Viral infection, heredity	Obesity, heredity, aging
Insulin required?	Yes	Sometimes
Cell response to insulin	Normal	Resistant
Symptoms	Relatively severe	Relatively moderate
Prevalence in diabetic	5% to 10%	90% to 95%

Source: Nutrition for Health & Health Care

USEFUL TERMS

Diabetes-related terms that are important in understanding and counseling African American patients.

50/50 Insulin:
Premixed insulin that is fifty percent (50%) intermediate acting (NPH) insulin and fifty percent (50%) short-acting or regular insulin.

70/30 Insulin:
Premixed insulin that is seventy percent (70%) intermediate acting [NPH] insulin and thirty percent (30%) short-acting or regular insulin.

A1C:
Also called glycosylated hemoglobin or hemoglobin A1C is a test that measures a person's average blood glucose level over the past 2 to 3 months. The test shows the amount of glucose that sticks to the red blood cell, which is proportional to the amount of glucose in the blood.

ACE Inhibitor:
An oral medicine that lowers blood pressure; Ace stands for 'angiotensin converting enzyme'. For people with diabetes, especially those who have protein (albumin) in the urine, it also helps slow down kidney damage.

Aspartame:
A dietary sweetener with almost no calories and no nutritional value. (Brand names; Equal, NutraSweet)

Blood Glucose:
The main sugar found in the blood and the body's main source of energy. Also called Blood sugar.

Blood Glucose level:
The amount of glucose in a given amount of blood. It is noted in milligrams in a deciliter, or mg/dl.

Blood Urea Nitrogen (BUN):
A waste product in the blood from the breakdown of protein. The kidneys filter blood to remove urea. As kidney function decreases, the BUN levels increase.

Body Mass Index (BMI):
A measure used to evaluate body weigh relative to a person's height. BMI is used to find out if a person is underweight, normal weight, overweight or obese.

Borderline Diabetes:
A former term for Type 2 diabetes or impaired glucose tolerance.

Brittle Diabetes:
A term used when a person's blood glucose level moves often from low to high and from high to low.

Carbohydrate Counting:
A method of meal planning for people with diabetes based on counting the number of grams of carbohydrate in food.

Creatinine:
A waste product from protein in the diet and from the muscles of the body. Creatinine is removed from the body by the kidney; as kidney disease progresses, the level of Creatinine in the blood increases.

Diabetic Ketoacidosis (DKA):
An emergency condition in which extremely high blood glucose levels, along with a severe lack of insulin, result in the breakdown of body fat for energy and an accumulation of ketones in the blood and urine. Signs of DKA are nausea and vomiting, stomach pain, fruity breath odor and rapid breathing. Untreated DKA can lead to coma and death.

Diabetic Nephropathy:
Disease of the kidney: Hyperglycemia and hypertension can damage the kidneys' glomeruli. When the kidneys are damaged, protein leaks out of the kidneys into the urine. Damaged kidneys can no longer remove waste and extra fluids from the bloodstream.

Diabetic Neuropathy:
Disease of the nervous system. The three major forms in people with diabetes are peripheral neuropathy, autonomic neuropathy, and mononeuropathy. The most common form is peripheral neuropathy, which affects mainly the legs and feet.

Diabetic Retinopathy:
Diabetic eye disease; damage to the small blood vessels in the retina. Loss of vision may result.

Exchange List:
One of several tools for diabetes meal planning. Foods are placed into three groups based on their nutritional content. Lists provide the serving sizes for carbohydrates, meat and meat alternatives and fats. These lists allow for substitution for different groups to keep the nutritional content fixed.

Fasting Blood Glucose Test:
A check of a person's blood glucose level after the person has not eaten for 8 to 12 hours (usually overnight). This test is used to diagnose pre-diabetes and diabetes. It is also used to monitor people with diabetes.

Gestational Diabetes Mellitus (GDM):
A type a diabetes mellitus that develops only during pregnancy and usually disappears upon delivery, but increases the risk that the mother will develop diabetes later. GDM is managed with meal planning, activity and, in some cases, insulin.

Glaucoma:
An increase in fluid pressure inside the eye that may lead to loss of vision.

Glycemic Index:
A ranking of carbohydrate-containing foods, based on the food's effect on blood glucose compared with a standard reference food.

Hyperglycemia:
Excessive blood glucose: Fasting hyperglycemia is blood glucose above a desirable level after a person has fasted for a least 8 hours. Postprandial hyperglycemia is blood glucose above a desirable level 1 to 2 hours after a person has eaten.

Hypoglycemia:
A condition that occurs when one's blood glucose is lower than normal, usually less than70mg/dl. Signs include hunger, nervousness, shakiness, perspiration, dizziness or light-headedness, sleepiness and confusion. If left untreated, hypoglycemia may lead to unconsciousness.

Juvenile Diabetes:
Former term for Insulin-dependent diabetes (IDDM), or Type 1 diabetes.

Ketone:
A chemical produced when there is a shortage of insulin the blood and the body breaks down body fat for energy. High levels of ketones can lead to diabetic Ketoacidosis and coma. Sometimes referred to as ketone bodies.

Urine testing:
Also called 'urinalysis'—A test of a urine sample to diagnose diseases of the urinary system and other body systems. Urine may also be checked for signs of bleeding. Some tests use a single urine sample. For others, 24-hour collection may be needed.

Xylitol:
A carbohydrate-based sweetener found in plants and used as a substitute for sugar; provides calories. Found in some mints and chewing gum.

Source: Adopted from Diabetes Information Library: Diabetes-Related Definitions

CHAPTER 3

DIETARY RECOMMENDATIONS

The medical nutrition therapy that is used as part of the management of diabetes mellitus is controlled in kilocalories (kcalories, but more often written as calories), proteins, fat and carbohydrate. The specific dietary recommendations or meal plan will vary with the type of diabetes mellitus and with the total medical management program as prescribed by the doctor or primary health care provider, and the registered dietitian.

KILOCALORIES

Following the American Diabetes Association guidelines:

12–20 % of kcalories should come from	-	protein
20–30 % of kcalories	-	fat
55–60 %	-	carbohydrate

to;
* achieve and maintain healthy body weight
* achieve normal growth and development
* to meet increased demands during pregnancy and lactation

CARBOHYDRATES

Following the American Diabetes Association guidelines:

55–60 % of kcalories should come from - carbohydrates

Although various starches have different glycemic responses, from a clinical perspective, the total amount of carbohydrate consumed is more important than the source of type of carbohydrate.

- individualized based on the persons eating habits
- distribution of carbohydrates in the meal pattern will vary with insulin regimens and treatment goals.

PROTEIN

Following the American Diabetes Association guidelines:

> 10–20 % of kcalories should come from -   protein

The RDA protein intake (0.8 g/kg body weight) for persons with diabetes is similar to non- diabetic persons.

FAT

Following the American Diabetes association guidelines:

> 20–30% of kilocalories should come from   - fat

note;

> < 10%   of kilocalories should come from   - saturated fat

> 60–70% of kilocalories should come from   - mono unsaturated fats

If obesity and weight loss are the primary concern, dietary fat intake must be reduced.

ALCOHOL

The consumption of Alcoholic beverages are not recommended for persons with diabetes. Like sugar, alcohol provides empty kcalories, and a high intake of alcoholic beverages may cause several health problems. Alcohol may have a hypoglycemic effect on persons with diabetes.

Simple alternatives may be club soda with lemon or lime, diet sodas or Perrier water.

CHAPTER 4

QUESTIONS ABOUT NUTRITION AND DIABETES

These are questions that the newly diagnosed diabetic may ask. The appropriate answers are provided.

Q. *Can I eat foods with sugar in them?*

A. Yes! The truth is that sugar has gotten a bad reputation. Eating a slice of cake with sugar will raise blood sugar levels but so will eating corn on the cob, a tomato sandwich or red (kidney) beans. In the body they are all converted to glucose and used for energy. With sugary foods, the rule is moderation.

Q. *Does losing weight help my diabetes?*

A. Yes! First, it lowers insulin resistance. This allows natural insulin to do a better job lowering blood glucose levels. Second, it improves blood fat and blood pressure levels, reducing the risk of cardiovascular disease.

Q. *How much weight should I lose each week?*

A. Limiting your weight loss to one pound a week will keep you healthy and will keep the weight off. The general rule is: the faster you take it off, the faster it comes back on. A slow steady weight loss is the key to keeping weight off.

Q. *What foods can I eat a lot of?*

A. The key to healthy living is moderation. If you can control the portion of the food you eat, you will be able to eat a wider variety of foods, including your favorites, and still stick to your goals.

Q.   *What can I do if I overeat over the holidays?*

A.   Put on your walking shoes and head for the pavement. Spend the extra holiday hours making sure you take a thirty or forty five minute walk, once a day to help lower blood glucose levels.

Q.   *Can I use all the artificial sweetener I want?*

A.   Artificial (calorie-free) sweeteners like aspartame, saccharin, and ace-sulfame-K won't increase blood glucose level. These sweeteners are safe for everyone except pregnant or breastfeeding women, who should not use saccharin, and people with phenylketonuria, who should not use aspartame.

Q.   *Can I drink alcohol?*

A.   Yes, in moderation. Moderation is defined as two drinks a day for men and one drink a day for women. A drink is a 5-ounce glass of wine, a 12-ounce light beer, or 1-1/2 ounces of 80-proof distilled spirits. Make sure that the medications that you are currently taking **do not** recommend avoiding alcohol, and get your doctor's okay.

Q.   *Isn't glucose control easier if I eat the same things every day?*

A.   Probably, but it can become boring and it may not be nutritious. From a nutritional standpoint, it is best to eat a variety of foods each day. By testing your blood glucose about an hour after meals, you will soon be able to predict what foods, and combinations of foods, raise your blood glucose levels.

Q.   *What vitamins will help my diabetes?*

A.   If you eat nutritiously, choosing a variety of fruits, vegetables, grains and meat each day, you wouldn't need to take vitamin supplements because of diabetes.

Q.   *Are there herbs that will help my diabetes?*

A.   Many herbs supposedly have glucose-lowering effects, but there are not enough data on any herb to recommend it for use in people with diabetes.

Q.   *Why do I need to see a dietitian?*

A.   Registered dietitians (RDs) have training and expertise in diabetes education and management, and are skilled in the coordination of diabetes medications and the diet. The RD will work with you to create a healthy eating plan that includes your favorite foods.

Source: Adapted from American Diabetes Association; Nutrition FAQs

CHAPTER 5

DIET—DRUG INTERACTIONS

Medications (also called Drugs) can be used to help control blood pressure. These oral antidiabetic agents must not be used to replace diet and physical activity in the management of diabetes. Patients must be advised to continue their medical nutritional therapy. People with type 1 diabetes need to utilize insulin to control blood glucose while people with type 2 diabetes need to utilize a combination of diet and physical activity to maintain blood pressure within normal limits. Oral antidiabetic medications are taken by mouth to assist with the lowering of blood glucose levels in people with type 2 diabetes.

The effects of drugs on the diet of the diabetic patient are often subtle, slow to appear and at times, hard to recognize. Foods can make a medication more or less powerful, and drugs can interfere with the body's ability to absorb nutrients from food. Drugs may also affect nutrition by causing loss of appetite, dry mouth, nausea, diarrhea or constipation.

The list below contains information about common interactions that may occur between food and drugs that may be taken for diabetes. It does not attempt to discuss all possible food-drug interactions, nor does it list possible drug-drug interactions.

Diet-Drug Interactions

Insulin:
The timing of *insulin* administration varies, depending on the Action of the insulin prescribed. Insulin may cause hypoglycemia.

Alpha-Glucosidase Inhibitors (Acarbose and Meglitol):
Alpha-Glucosidase Inhibitors are taken at the start of each meal. Clients using these agents must use glucose to treat hypoglycemia. Nutrition-related side effects include abdominal pain, gas and diarrhea.

Lispro (Insulin Analog):
Lispro is taken 5 to 10 minutes before meals. Lispro lowers The risk of hypoglycemia compared to insulin.

Metformin:
Metformin is taken once or twice a day before meals (breakfast or breakfast and dinner). GI side effects are uncommon, but metformin may cause diarrhea or leave a metallic taste in the mouth.

Nateglinide:
Nateglinide is taken immediately before eating. Nateglinide can cause hypoglycemia and sometimes diarrhea.

Repaglinide:
Repaglinide is taken before meals. Repaglinide can cause hypoglycemia and diarrhea.

Sulfonylureas
(Chlorpropamide, Glipzide, Glyburide, Glimepiride):
Sulfonylureas are generally taken one or two times a day, before Meals. Disulfiram-like reactions can occur when large amounts of alcohol are taken (especially with chlorpropamide). These medications can also cause hypoglycemia.

Thioglitazones
(Rosiglitazone, Piolitazone):
Thioglitazones are taken once or twice a day before meals. Nutrition Related side effects are uncommon. One medication of this type, Troglitazone, was recently taken off the market due to concerns that its Use might be a cause of liver failure.

Source: Adapted from "Understanding Normal and Clinical Nutrition" sixth Edition.

CHAPTER 6

GENERAL PROTOCOL
FOR
IDDM OR TYPE1 DIABETES

GOAL:

To maintain day-to-day consistency in the timing and amount of food intake in persons receiving conventional Insulin therapy.

GUIDELINES:

* **Consume adequate kilocalories to maintain healthy weight.**
(Kilocalorie [kcalorie] intake for the meal plan should be determined by the primary healthcare provider. example: MD, RN or RD. Whenever possible, the dietitian RD, should provide diet instructions.)

* **Keep the timing of meals consistent from day to day, and synchronized with the time-actions of insulin.**
It is not necessary to provide meals and snacks into any artificial or unnatural division. Stay as close as possible to the usually eating pattern of the individual.

* **Depending upon the insulin regimen, plan a bedtime snack to prevent nocturnal hypoglycemia.**

EXAMPLE OF DAILY MEAL PLAN:

If an individual is receiving conventional Insulin therapy;

3 meals per day   (spaced 4-5 hours apart)
bedtime snack

therefore;

Inject AM insulin   ½ hour before breakfast
Other insulin   ½ hour before meal
Or at designated evening time

Usually only 15 gm of carbohydrate (1 starch exchange), and 1 oz of protein (1 exchange) are needed for a bedtime snack.

Example of 15 gm carbohydrate: -

4 ozs. apple/orange juice
10 ozs. milk
3 graham crackers
6 saltine crackers
3 glucose tablets
4 life savers (hard candy)

Example of 1 ounce protein:-

8 ozs. milk
1 carton yogurt
  (w/NutraSweet)
1 oz. Cheese
1 egg
2 Tablespoons Peanut butter

* Limit simple carbohydrate to 10%–15 of total kcalories

Simple Carbohydrates: defined as mono and disaccharides
which are lactose, sucrose and fructose.

Example: Table sugar
Corn syrup
Honey
Molasses

* Make modifications in the dietary management plan for hypertension, hyperlipidemia and/or renal insufficiency.
Eat salt and sodium in moderation. Do not advise the use of any commercially prepared or seasoned meats, entrees, vegetables, potatoes, macaroni or rice dishes.

Limit fried foods to only one time every other week (biweekly). Fats, such as margarine mayonnaise, salad dressings should be used sparingly -1 teaspoon/per serving.

* If obesity or overweight is present, follow a low kcalorie diet to reduce and maintain a desirable weight.
Regular exercise is of primary importance in achieving desirable weight.

NOTE: Advise all patients to consult a doctor before starting any exercise regime.

* Test blood glucose 2–4 times daily.

TREATMENT FOR HYPOGLYCEMIA

If Hypoglycemia occurs the 15:15 Rule should be applied

RULE:

TAKE 15 GRAMS OF FAST ACTING SUGAR
WAIT 15 MINUTES THEN CHECK BLOOD LEVELS
IF GREATER THAN 70 MG %—EAT SNACK OR MEAL
BUT;
IF LESS THAN 70 MG %—REPEAT THE 15:15 RULE

********* 15 Grams of carbohydrate should increase blood
sugar by 30 mg % in 15 minutes ********

CHAPTER 7

GENERAL PROTOCOL
FOR
NIDDM OR TYPE 11 DIABETES

GOAL:

To follow an appropriate dietary regime, that will best achieve a satisfactory (acceptable) blood glucose levels.

GUIDELINES:

*   Eat well- balanced meals, including: Protein, Starch, Vegetables and Fruit.

Example: 3ozs. meat	=	the size of a deck of cards
starches	=	rice, potatoes, breads, and starchy vegetables <u>ex.</u> beans, peas, and corn
vegetables	=	broccoli, green beans, cabbage, carrots
fruits	=	fresh, canned fruit or juice.

* **Keep the timing of the meals and the composition of the diet consistent from day to day.**
Spread the nutrients throughout the day, instead of only in three meals.

When eating fruit or drinking fruit juice, always have it with a meal or snack, never on an empty stomach. REMEMBER ; never drink more than 4 ozs. (1/2 cup) of juice at one time.

* A kilocalorie-restricted diet (sometimes referred to as a low calorie diet) must be followed if obesity is present.
Rule of Thumb:
A moderate kcalorie- restricted diet is one that has 250-500 kcalories less daily, than the usual daily intake.

* Limit simple carbohydrate to 10%–15% of the total kcalories
Simple Carbohydrates: defined as mono., and disaccharides

which are lactose, sucrose and fructose.
Example: table sugar
Corn syrup
Honey
Molasses
Sorghum

* The carbohydrate content (bread exchange) should be evenly divided from meal to meal
Avoid concentrated sweets: candy, colas, doughnuts, ketchup etc.

Drink diet beverages only: Use an artificial sweetener in coffee, tea or lemonade etc.

* Regular exercise is of primary importance in achieving desirable weight.
Even a moderate weight loss (10-20 pounds) has been shown to improve diabetes control.

NOTE: Consult a doctor before starting any exercise regime.

*Plan a bedtime snack to prevent nocturnal hypoglycemia when either a short or long acting hypoglycemia agent is used. (chlorpropamide, glyburide, acetohexamide, tolbutamide, tolazamide, glipzide etc.)

Usually only 15 gm of carbohydrate (1starch exchange), and 1 oz of protein (1 exchange) are needed for a bedtime snack.

Example of 15 gm carbohydrate:-	4	ozs. apple/orange juice
	10	ozs. milk
	3	grahams crackers
	5	saltine crackers
	6	glucose tablets
	7	life savers (hard candy)
Example of 1 ounce protein:-	8	ozs. milk
	1	carton yogurt (w/NutraSweet)
	1	oz. Cheese
	1	egg
	2	tablespoons Peanut butter

* Test blood glucose 2-4 times daily.

TREATMENT FOR HYPOGLYCEMIA

If Hypoglycemia occurs the 15:15 Rule should be applied

RULE:

TAKE 15 GRAMS OF FAST ACTING SUGAR
WAIT 15 MINUTES THEN CHECK BLOOD LEVELS
IF GREATER THAN 70 MG %—EAT SNACK OR MEAL BUT;
IF LESS THAN 70 MG %—REPEAT THE 15: 15 RULE

******** 15 Grams of carbohydrate should increase blood sugar by 30 mg % in 15 minutes. ***********

Modifications in the "Soul Food Diet" in NIDDM

The traditional diet of most African Americans follow closely the 'traditional soul food diet' which utilized fried foods, saturated fat and high-fat products, exacerbating obesity and the risk factors for diabetes.

The information provided below is useful when counseling the African American patient.

General recommendations:

The amount and type of fat must be modified to encourage healthy kcaloric intake and to prevent the risk of obesity, and associated health factors. Correct portion sizes must be strictly maintained, and the consumption of a meatless main dish at least twice per week, should be encouraged, to promote healthy weight. Emphasize the benefits of whole grain products, fresh fruits and vegetables and the use of acceptable alternative sweeteners.

Foods to be avoided:	Foods that can be used:
High-fat meats;	
Chicken wings	Vegetables oil
Bologna	skin-free turkey necks
Sausages	liquid smoke (for flavor)
Fried Meats	margarine
Lard	egg whites
Ham hocks	fat-free broth
Bacon grease	
White bread	whole wheat, whole grain bread
Cakes	whole wheat pasta
Pies	beans, peas
White (flour) pasta	sugar-free dessert products
Soft drinks	Soft drinks
Ice Cream	Ice cream
	Yogurt
	Pudding
	Cake

Source: Modified from 'Ethnic and regional Food practices: Soul and Traditional Southern Food Practices, Customs, and Holiday'

CHAPTER 8

CARBOHYDRATE COUNTING

During the past decade a paradigm shift has occurred in Diabetes Management. Priority is being given to *the total amount of carbohydrate* consumed at each meal and at snack time, rather than the *source* of the carbohydrate. When an individual with diabetes has the ability to control their daily carbohydrate intake, they are better able to manage their blood glucose levels. Carbohydrates affect the glucose levels in blood more than protein or fat.

To be competent with carbohydrate counting, patients must first understand the exchange list system and establish healthy eating habits, use correct portion sizes, and learn to eat a consistent amount of carbohydrate at regular times. Where possible the services of a dietitian or nutritionist should be used because they are the best trained health care professional to offer assistance with calculating the carbohydrates and calories that are appropriate for each diabetic patient.

RULE of THUMB:

About half (50%) of the kcalories intake should be carbohydrates (carbs). There are about 4 calories in every gram of carbohydrates.

REMEMBER

Example:
With a meal plan of 1200 calories a day
About 600 calories should be from carbohydrates
600 divided by 4   = 150 carb grams daily
Daily goal   = 150 grams

Formula:
(calories/2)/4   = carb grams per day

Once the goal for carbohydrate is established it becomes essential that the diabetic individual learns to determine the amount of carbohydrates in various portion sizes of food. Routine use of the *Food Facts Label*, and using the *Exchange List for Meal Planning* will help to determine and monitor total carbohydrate intake.

Remember:
When using the exchange system, one starch exchange equals about 15 grams of carbohydrate. One milk exchange is about 12 grams, and a vegetable exchange is about 15 grams.

To use this system effectively the common measuring units used by the patient must be reviewed and completely understood.

COMMON MEASUREMENTS:

3 teaspoons (tsp.)	=	1 tablespoon (Tbsp.)
4 tablespoons (Tbsps.)	=	¼ cup
5 1/3 tablespoons (Tbsps.)	=	1/3 cup
4 ounces (ozs.)	=	½ cup
8 ounces (ozs.)	=	1 cup
1 cup	=	½ pint

The advantages of this technique include more precise matching of food and insulin, greater flexibility with food choices, and an improved potential for success with food intake and improved blood glucose control.

CHAPTER 9

THE GLYCEMIC INDEX

The glycemic index is another tool that is useful in the teaching and counseling of the diabetic patients. The index measures how fast a food item is likely to raise blood sugar levels, and therefore can be helpful for managing sugars levels in the blood. The glycemic index is an indicator of the 'after-meal' response that the body has to a particular food compared to the reference standard, glucose; the fastest absorbed carbohydrate available. Glucose is given the value of one hundred (100) on the glycemic index, and other carbohydrates are given a number or an index relative to glucose.

Foods with a high glycemic index raise blood glucose faster and to a greater extent than foods with a low glycemic index. For example, if blood sugar levels tend to drop rapidly during exercise the consumption of a carbohydrate food that will raise blood sugar quickly (high glycemic index) is suggested. On the other hand, to help keep the blood sugar level as constant as possible during a few hours of mild activity, the consumption of a carbohydrate food that will raise blood sugar more slowly (lower glycemic index) is suggested. Carbohydrate foods with a lower glycemic index, also called slower carbs, are helpful for preventing overnight drops in the sugar level of the blood, and for long periods of exercise.

Since people are individuals and respond differently to metabolic changes, registered dietitians often encourage patients to monitor their blood sugar responses to carbohydrates foods, thereby creating their own individual glycemic index.

The Glycemic Index Range and a list of common carbohydrate foods with the corresponding index is provided below:

Glycemic Index Range

Low Glycemic Index	=	55 or less
Medium Glycemic Index	=	56–69
High Glycemic Index	=	70 or more

****REMEMBER:**

The glycemic index is an additional tool that works together with the patient's current meal planning system to successfully control daily blood glucose (sugar) levels.

Glycemic Index Guide : Examples of Foods by Categories

FOOD CATEGORIES	INDEX	FOOD CATEGORIES	INDEX
CEREALS		**FRUIT**	
All Bran	51	Apple	38
Cheerios	74	Banana	56
Cornflakes	83	Grapefruit	25
Life	66	Mango	55
Oatmeal, old fashion	48	Peach	42
Raisin Bran	73	Watermelon	72
SNACKS		**CRACKERS**	
Chocolate Bar	49	Graham crackers	74
Croissant	67	Rice cakes	80
Doughnut	76	Pretzels	83
Pizza Hut, supreme	33	Soda crackers, saltines	72
Pound Cake	54	Wheat thins	67
Oatmeal Cookies	55	Rye	68
GRAINS		**SUGARS/CANDIES**	
Barley	25	Fructose	22
Basmati white Rice	58	Honey	62
Brown Rice	55	Table sugar (sucrose)	64
Instant White Rice	87	Glucose Tablets	102
Couscous	65	Jelly Beans	80
Cornmeal	68	M&M chocolate candies	33
PASTA		**VEGETABLES**	
Fettuccini	32	Carrot	49
Macaroni	45	Green Pea	47
Macaroni and Cheese Dinner	64	Lima Beans	32
Spaghetti	33	Corn	56
Cheese Tortellini	50	Parsnips	97
Vermicelli	35	Tomato	38

FOOD CATEGORIES	INDEX	FOOD CATEGORIES	INDEX
BEANS/ROOT CROPS		BREADS	
Baked beans	48	Bagel, plain	72
Kidney beans	52	Croissant	67
Black beans	30	Blueberry muffin	59
Chickpeas (garbanzo beans)	33	White, sliced	70
Sweet potatoes	54	Whole wheat	68
White potatoes (Irish)	70	Pumpernickel, whole grain	49
DRINKS		MILK PRODUCTS	
Apple juice	40	Whole milk	30
Colas (sodas)	65	Chocolate milk	35
Gatorade	78	Skim milk	32
Grapefruit juice	48	Soy milk	31
Orange juice	46	Ice cream	60
Pineapple juice	46	Yogurt, fruit	36

Steps To Incorporating a Low Glycemic Index Diet

The use of the glycemic index meal-planning tool can be introduced to the patient through a series of recommendations. Recommend that patients;

· Use breakfast cereals based on oats, barley and bran
· Use 'grainy' bread made with whole seeds
· Reduce the amount of potatoes eaten
· Enjoy all types of fruit and vegetables (except potatoes)
· Eat plenty of salad vegetables with vinaigrette dressing

Source: modified from Home of the Glycemic Index. www.glycemicindex.com; and Food and Diet in Diabetes. www.Diabetesnet.com

CHAPTER 10

MEAL PLAN

The Meal Plan is the primary tool used by most RDs and other health professionals to teach diabetic patients how to best manage their dietary plan.

The meal is a guide that shows the number of food choices or exchanges available at each meal and at snack time.

NOTE:

> IT IS RECOMMENDED THAT A DIETITIAN OR NUTRITIONIST DESIGN THE MEAL PLAN BASED ON INDIVIDUAL NEEDS.

MEAL PLANS:

The table below shows sample meal plans for different kilocalorie levels. The kilocaloric levels are usually prescribed by the attending doctor.

	1,200	1,500	1,800	2,000	2,500	Other:
Carbohydrates	(11)	(13)	(16)	(17)	(22)	
Starch	5	7	8	9	11	
Fruit	3	3	4	4	6	
Milk	2	2	3	3	3	
Vegetables	2	2	3	4	5	
Other						
Meat & Meat Substitutes	4	4	6	6	8	
Fat	3	4	4	5	6	

Explanation:

The numbers that are displayed throughout the table reflect the number of exchanges (measured portions) from each food group available daily on a specific meal plan.

A 1,200 kcalorie meal plan has 11 exchanges of carbohydrates. This includes 5 exchanges from starch, 3 from fruit, 2 from milk and 2 from starchy vegetables. Four (4) exchanges will come from meat and 3 exchanges will come from fat.

Example of Sample Menu for a day

This is a 1,200 kcalorie meal plans with 10-11 carbohydrate exchanges.

Breakfast:	1 scrambled egg
	1 buttermilk biscuit (1)
	1 tsp. margarine
	½ grapefruit section (1)
	8 fl. oz. skim milk (1)

Lunch:	1 cup macaroni & cheese (2)
	½ cup carrot sticks
	½ cup celery sticks
	2 Tbsp. dip
	1 cup melon (1)
	diet soda

Dinner:	½ cup red beans and rice (1)
	2 ozs cornbread (1)
	½ cup cooked greens
	1 tsp. olive oil
	½ cup canned peaches (1)
	8 fl. ozs skim milk (1)

Source: adapted from 'Eating Right When You Have Diabetes'.

CHAPTER 11

THE FOOD EXCHANGE LIST

WHAT ARE THE EXCHANGE LISTS?

They are lists of foods that are grouped together because they have about the same amount of carbohydrate, protein fat and kcalories. In the amounts given, any food on a list can be exchanged, traded or swapped for any other food on the same list. Several foods, such as beans and peas are on two lists.

The complete listing of the United States Exchange Lists can be obtained for patient use, from the web site of the American Dietetic Association and the American Diabetic Association.

Example of the Exchange list

VEGETABLES:
Contain 25 calories and 5 grams of carbohydrates. One serving equals:

½ cup	Cooked vegetables (carrots, broccoli, zucchini, cabbage)
1 cup	Raw vegetables or salad greens
½ cup	Vegetable Juice

FAT-FREE and LOWFAT MILK:
Contain 90 calories. One serving equals:

1 cup	Milk, fat-free or 1% fat
¾ cup	Yogurt, plain non fat or low fat
1 cup	Yogurt, artificially sweetened

VERY LEAN PROTEIN:
Contain 35 calories and 1 gram fat per serving. One serving equals:

1 ounce	Turkey or Chicken breast
1 ounce	Fisk fillet
1 ounce	Canned tuna in water
1 ounce	Shellfish (clams, lobster, scallop, shrimp)
¾ cup	Cottage cheese, non fat or low fat
2 each	Egg whites
¼ cup	Egg substitute
1 ounce	Fat-free cheese
½ cup	Beans—cooked (black beans, kidney, chick peas or lentils): count as 1 starch/bread and 1 very lean protein.

LEAN PROTEIN:
Contains 55 calories and 2-3 grams of fat per serving. One serving equals:

1 ounce	Chicken—dark meat
1 ounce	Turkey—dark meat
1 ounce	Salmon, Swordfish, Herring
1 ounce	Lean beef
1 ounce	Veal, Roast or Lean chop*
1 ounce	Lamb, Roast or Lean chop*
1 ounce	Pork, tenderloin or fresh ham*
¼ cup	4.5% cottage cheese
2 medium	Sardines

(*Limit to 1-2 times per week)

MEDIUM FAT PROTEINS:
Contains 75 calories and 5 grams of fat per serving. One serving equals:

1 ounce	Beef (any prime cut), corned beef, ground beef**
1 ounce	Pork chop
1 each	Whole egg (medium)**
1 ounce	Mozzarella cheese
¼ cup	Ricotta cheese
4 ounces	Tofu

(**Choose these very infrequently)

FRUITS:

Contain 15 grams of carbohydrates and 60 calories. One serving equals:

1 small	Apple, banana, orange, nectarine
1 medium	Fresh peach
1	Kiwi
½	Grapefruit
½	Mango
1 cup	Fresh berries (strawberries, raspberries or blueberries)
1 cup	Fresh melon cubes
1/8th	Honeydew melon
4 ounces	Unsweetened Juice
4 teaspoons	Jelly or Jam

STARCHES:

Contains 15 grams of carbohydrate and 80 calories. One serving equals:

1 slice	Bread (white, pumpernickel, whole wheat, rye)
2 slice	Reduced calorie or 'lite' Bread
¼ (1 ounce)	Bagel
½	English muffin
½	Hamburger bun
¾ cup	cold cereal
1/3 cup	Rice, brown or white
1/3 cup	Barley or Couscous
1/3 cup	Legumes
½ cup	pasta

FATS

Contains 45 calories and 5 grams fat per serving. One serving equals:

1 teaspoon	Oil (vegetable, corn, canola, olive etc.)
1 teaspoon	Butter
1 teaspoon	Stick margarine
1 teaspoon	Mayonnaise
1 Tablespoon	Salad dressing
1 slice	Bacon
1/8th	Avocado

Source: Food Exchange List—National Institute of Health [adapted from ADA Exchange List]

RECIPES FOR THE AFRICAN AMERICAN PALATE

The recipes in this section are teaching tools,
and may be
used as handouts for the patients.

CHAPTER 12

FAVORITE DIABETIC RECIPES

Hot Garlic Shrimp

Source: The Diabetes Double-Quick Cookbook
Author: Betty Marks

1 pound large shrimp
1 tbsp olive oil
4 cloves garlic, smashed, peeled or minced
1/2 to 1 tsp red pepper flakes
dash cumin
3 tbsp lemon juice
parsley, chopped, for garnish

Peel and devein shrimp and rinse in cold water. Mix olive oil and garlic in glass measuring cup and microwave on high for 1 minute. In a 2-quart round casserole, mix shrimp with oil and garlic, and sprinkle with red pepper, a few dashes of cumin, and lemon juice. Stir to mix and arrange shrimp in circular fashion, thick ends to the outside of bowl. Cover with vented plastic wrap and microwave on high for 3 to 4 minutes, turning shrimp once. Remove when shrimp are pink. Let stand another minute to complete cooking. Dust with parsley.

Makes 4 Serving   *Dietary Exchanges: 3 Lean Meat*

Nutrients per Serving:
156 Calories   5 g Fat   0.8 g Saturated Fat 1.1 g Polyunsaturated Fat
174 mg Cholesterol 24 g Protein 0 g Dietary Fiber   2.8 g Monounsaturated Fat
3 g Carbohydrate   171 mg Sodium

Barbecued Chicken

Source: Diabetic Recipes

3 lbs. chicken pieces

1 small onion

1/2 cup tomato sauce

1/2 cup nonfat plain yogurt

1 tsp. fresh ginger, chopped

2 garlic cloves

2 tsp. coriander

1/2 tsp. cayenne pepper (optional)

2 whole cloves

1 tsp. cumin seeds

4 cardamom pods

1 tsp. salt

Remove the skin and all visible fat from the chicken pieces. (I often have the butcher skin the chicken.) Cut 2-3 slits, 1 inch long and 1/2 inch deep, in each piece of chicken. Place in a casserole dish and set aside. Cut onion into 4-5 pieces. In a blender jar put onion, tomato sauce, yogurt, ginger, garlic cloves, coriander, cayenne pepper, cloves, cumin seeds and salt. Blend to a smooth paste. Pour the paste on the chicken and turn pieces to thoroughly coat with spices. Cover with a lid or plastic wrap and marinate in the refrigerator 4-24 hours. Preheat oven to 400°F. Remove chicken pieces from the marinade, saving marinade. Arrange pieces in a broiler pan. Bake uncovered in the middle of the oven for 30 minutes. Turn pieces over and brush with remaining marinade. Bake for 10-15 minutes until chicken is tender. Turn oven to broil. Turn pieces over once again and broil for 5 minutes. Transfer to a serving platter. Serve with lemon wedges or squeeze lemon juice over the chicken before eating, if desired.

Per serving: calories 293, fat 7.2g, 23% calories from fat, cholesterol 159mg, protein 50.2g, carbohydrates 4.3g, fiber 0.6g, sodium 551mg

Sweet and Sour Chicken Salad

Source: Diabetic Recipes

1-1/4 lbs. boneless skinless chicken breast, cooked and cut into 2 inch cubes

1-1/2 cups celery, diagonally sliced

1 cup snow peas, trimmed

1/2 cup red bell pepper, seeded and diced

1 cup apples, peeled and diced

1/4 cup vinegar

1/4 cup vegetable oil

2 Tbs. sugar

1 tsp. paprika

1 tsp. celery seed

salt and pepper, to taste

Combine all salad ingredients. Whisk together the dressing ingredients. Pour the dressing over the salad and serve.

Per serving: calories 249, fat 12.0g, 43% calories from fat, cholesterol 60mg, protein 23.1g, carbohydrates 12.6g, fiber 2.0g, sodium 81mg.

Exchanges: 1 Carbohydrate, 3 Lean Meat, 1/2 Monosaturated Fat.

Diabetic Homemade Ice Cream

Source: Diabetic Recipes

13 ounces evaporated milk

2 Tbsp. sugar replacement

1-1/2 cup whole milk

1 Tbsp. vanilla extract

3 eggs (well beaten)

Combine evaporated milk and sugar replacement. Beat well until sugar is dissolved. Add whole milk and vanilla extract; beat well. Add eggs; beat eggs into milk mixture vigorously. Pour into ice cream maker. Freeze according to manufacturer's directions.

1 serving = 1/2 milk, 1/2 lean meat Calories = 122

Sole Almondine

Source: The Diabetes Double-Quick Cookbook
Author: Betty Marks

1-2 tbsp butter

2-4 tbsp slivered blanched almonds

1 tbsp chopped parsley

2 tbsp dry white wine

1/4 c chicken broth

2 sole fillets (or flounder) about 6 ounces each

Heat 1 tablespoon of butter on high in an 8-inch square browning pan a few seconds. Add almonds and parsley and stir to blend. Cook on high for one minute. Remove dish from oven, add wine and chicken broth, and place fish in center of dish. Cover with plastic wrap and microwave on high for 2 1/2 minutes. Uncover and place on serving dish, whisking remaining butter into almond sauce. Serve with asparagus and light grain.

Makes 2 Servings   *Dietary Exchanges: 2 Meat, 1 Fat*

Nutrients per Serving:
179 Calories, 15 g Protein, 11 g Fat, 221mg. Sodium, 4.3 g Saturated Fat
4.8 g Monounsaturated Fat, 1.1 g Dietary Fiber, 51.5 mg Cholesterol

Banana French Toast

Source: Heart Smart Cookbook

1 whole egg, slightly beaten

2 egg whites

1 tablespoon honey

¼ teaspoon cinnamon

¼ cup skim milk

1 mashed, overripe banana

Vegetable cooking spray

10 slices whole wheat bread

Heat griddle or skillet to medium heat. In a shallow bowl or pie pan, mix egg, egg whites, honey, cinnamon, milk and banana.

Spray vegetable cooking spray onto the griddle. Dip bread in the egg mixture, turning to coat both sides. Cook on griddle, about 4 minutes on each side or until golden brown.

Makes 5 serving.   *Dietary Exchanges: 2 starch, ½ fat*

Nutrition Information per Serving:
187 Calories,   4g Fat, 8g Protein, 359 mg. Sodium, trace Saturated fat,
*   55 mg. Cholesterol*

Southern Black-Eyed Peas

Source: Heart Smart Cookbook

2 cups Shelled fresh or frozen black-eyed peas

2 cups water

Vegetable Spray

1 medium chopped onion

½ teaspoon beef-flavored bouillon granules

¼ teaspoon ground savory

¼ teaspoon crushed red pepper flakes

If you use fresh peas, wash and drain them well. Combine peas and water in a medium saucepan; bring to a boil. Cover, reduce heat and simmer for 10 minutes. Meanwhile, spray a medium nonstick skillet with vegetable cooking spray, about 3 minutes. Add bouillon granules, savory and red pepper flakes and stir to combine. Add onion mixture to beans, cover and let simmer 50 minutes more or until tender.

Makes 4 servings   *Dietary exchanges;;1 starch, 1 vegetable*

Nutrition Information per serving:
104 calories,	*1 g Fat,*	*0g Saturated fat,*	*trace Cholesterol*
154 mg Sodium,	*7g Protein,*	*17g Carbohydrate*	

Cajun-Style Catfish

Source: Heart Smart Cookbook

1-1/2 cups fresh orange juice

2 tablespoons fresh lemon juice

3 tablespoons fresh lime juice

1 tablespoon rice vinegar

3 cloves garlic, peeled, ends removed

2 tablespoons jalapeno peppers, seeded & diced (optional)

¼ cup chili powder

¼ teaspoon black pepper

1 pound catfish

Preheat grill or broiler.
In a medium bowl combine orange juice, lemon juice, lime juice, rice vinegar, garlic, jalapeno peppers (optional), chili powder, and black pepper.
Arrange each fish filet on a sheet of aluminum foil. Bring edges of foil upwards to form a bowl. Spoon 2 tablespoons of sauce over each fillet. Pinch top edges of foil together, leaving a small amount of space for steam to escape.
Arrange foil packets on a grill and cook 8 to 10 minutes, or until fish flakes easily when tested with a fork. Heat remaining sauce and serve with fish.

Makes 4 servings.   *Dietary Exchanges: 3 lean meat, 1 fruit*

Nutrition Information per serving:
185 calories,	*5g Fat,*	*1g Saturated fat,*	*45mg Cholesterol*
126 mg Sodium,	*24g Protein,*	*17g Carbohydrate*	

Sugar-Free Sweet Potato Pie

Source: Calorie Control Council

2-1/2 cups Mashed cooked Sweet Potatoes

¼ tsp. Ground mace

1 Tbsp. Softened margarine

2 tsp. Ground cinnamon

¾ tsp. Ground nutmeg

7-1/4 tsp. artificial sweetener (Equal, Splenda etc.)

2 tsp. vanilla extract

2 eggs

2 unbaked 9-inch pie shells

½ tsp. salt

1 (12 ounce) can evaporated skim milk

Preheat oven to 350 degrees.
In a large bowl combine the sweet potatoes, eggs, artificial sweetener, margarine, cinnamon, nutmeg, mace, salt and vanilla. Using an electric mixer, beat on medium speed until smooth, scraping the sides of the bowl several times. Slowly add milk. Beat until well mixed. Pour into unbaked pie shells and bake for 50 to 60 minutes or until the knife inserted in the center of pie, comes out clean. Allow to cool before serving.

Makes 16 servings (2; 9-inch pies)
Dietary Exchanges: 1 vegetable, 2 Breads, 2-1/2 Fat.

Nutrition Information per serving:
208 calories,   9g Fat,   27mg Cholesterol,   245mg Sodium

Breakfast Shake

Source: Calorie Control Council

½ cup low-fat yogurt

¼ cup skim milk

2 tablespoons frozen orange juice concentrate

2 packets artificial sweetener

3 ice cubes

1 tablespoon wheat germ

½ teaspoon vanilla extract

In a blender at medium speed, blend all ingredients until smooth and frothy. Pour into a glass and enjoy.

Variation: Add ½ cup sliced banana or strawberries: blend as directed

Makes 1-1/2 cups   *Dietary Exchanges: 1 bread, 1 fruit, 1 non-fat milk*

Nutrition Information per serving:
220 calories,   *10g Protein,*   *42g Carbohydrate*   *1g total Fat*
110 mg Sodium,   *< 1mg Cholesterol*

REFERENCES

African American Program. American Diabetes Association

Diabetes Among African Americans. American Diabetes Association www.diabetes.org/ada/facts . Retrieved (2004)

Diabetic Recipes. www.diabetessymptom.net Retrieved (2004)

Cataldo, C. B., DeBruyne, L. K., Whitney, E, N. *Nutrition and Diet Therapy: Principles and Practice.* Wadworth/Thomson Learning, 2003

Counting Calories and Carbs. Novo Nordisk Pharmaceuticals Inc., 1998

Ethnic and Regional Food Practices, A Series. *Soul and Traditional Southern Food Practices, Customs, and Holidays.* The American Dietetic Association, & The Diabetes Association, Inc. (1995)

Ewing, J., *Cultural Diversity: Eating in American, African American* HYG-5250-95 www.ohioline.osu.edu Retrieved (2004)

Food & Diet in Diabetes. *Glycemic Index. How quickly do foods raise your blood sugar?* www.diabetesnet.com Retrieved (2004)

Food and Drug Interactions. Munson Army Health Center. 2001 www.munson.amedd.army.mil. Retrieved (2004)

Frequently asked Questions: Nutrition and Diabetes. American Diabetes Association 2000. www.diabetes.org/nutirtion/faqs.asp. Retrieved (2004)

Heart Smart Cookbook. Henry Ford Heart & Vascular Institute and The Detroit Free Press. (1995)

Joslin Diabetes Center. *What is the Glycemic Index and Is It a Helpful Tool?* www.joslin.harvard.edu Retrieved (2004)

National Heart, Lung, and Blood Institute. *Food Exchange List*. www.nhlbi.nih.gov Retrieved (2004)

Powers, M., *Guide To Eating Right When You Have Diabetes; The Comprehensive approach to Managing your Diabetes by eating well*. American Dietetic Association 2003.

Recipes. Calorie Control Council 2000. www.caloriecontrol.org Retrieved (2004)

Single-Topic Diabetes Resources. The American Dietetic Association, & The Diabetes Association, Inc. (1995)

Whitney, E. N., Cataldo, C.B., Rolfes, S.R. *Understanding Normal and Clinical Nutrition*. Sixth Edition. Wadworth/Thomson Learning Inc. 2002.

ABOUT THE AUTHOR

Cheryl Campbell Atkinson PhD, RD., LDN.

Received her B.S. in Food Science and Management from Pratt Institute in Brooklyn New York in 1977, her M.P.H. in Nutrition from Tulane University in New Orleans, Louisiana and her Ph.D. in International Nutrition from Cornell University in 1993. She is a registered dietitian (RD) and a licensed dietitian/nutritionist (LDN), and a member of both the American Dietetic Association and the American Association of Family and Consumer Sciences. She has worked in private practice as a clinical dietitian in Baltimore, Maryland and New Orleans, Louisiana, and is presently a faculty member at Southern University A&M College, Baton Rouge, Louisiana.

0-595-32901-2

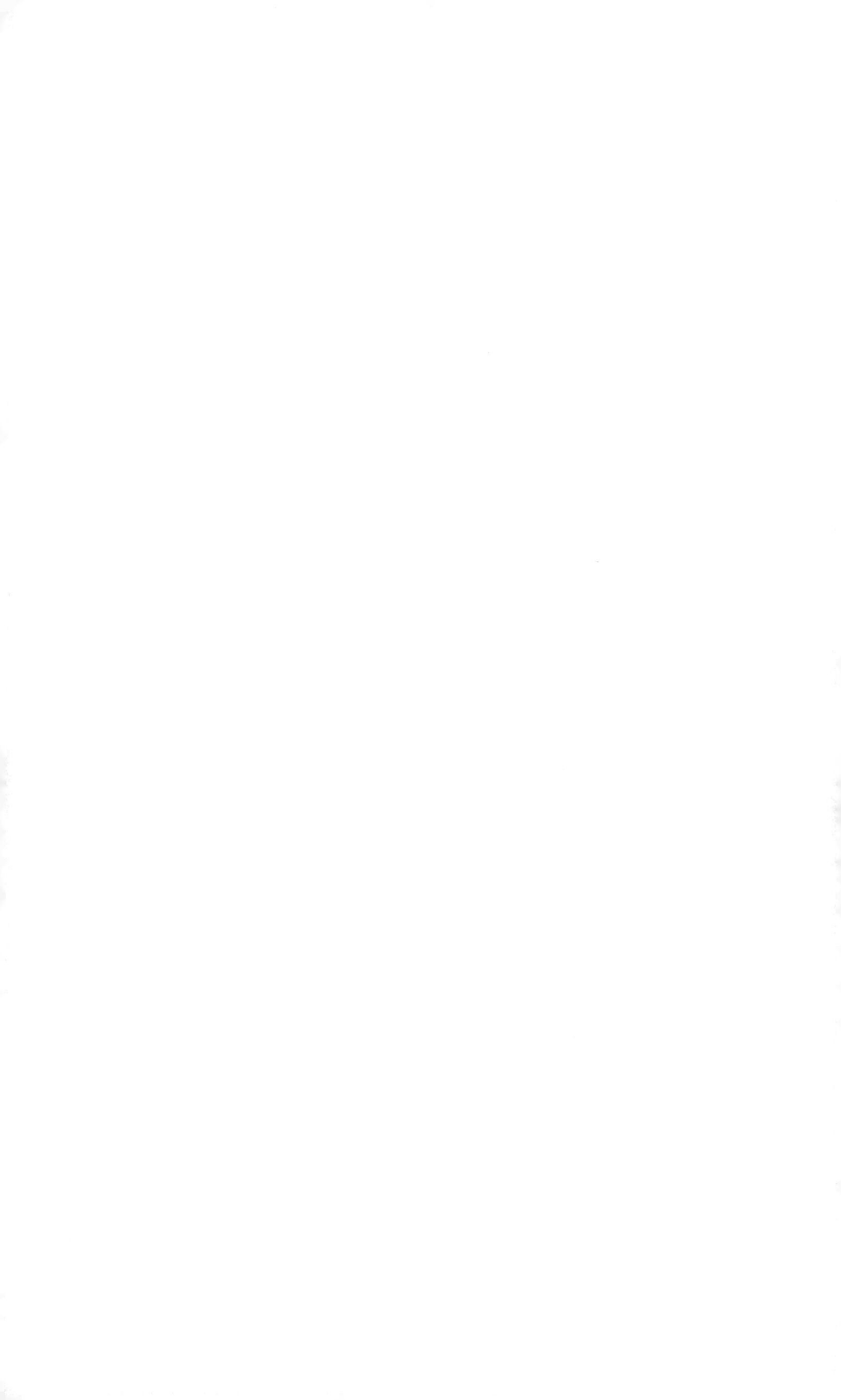

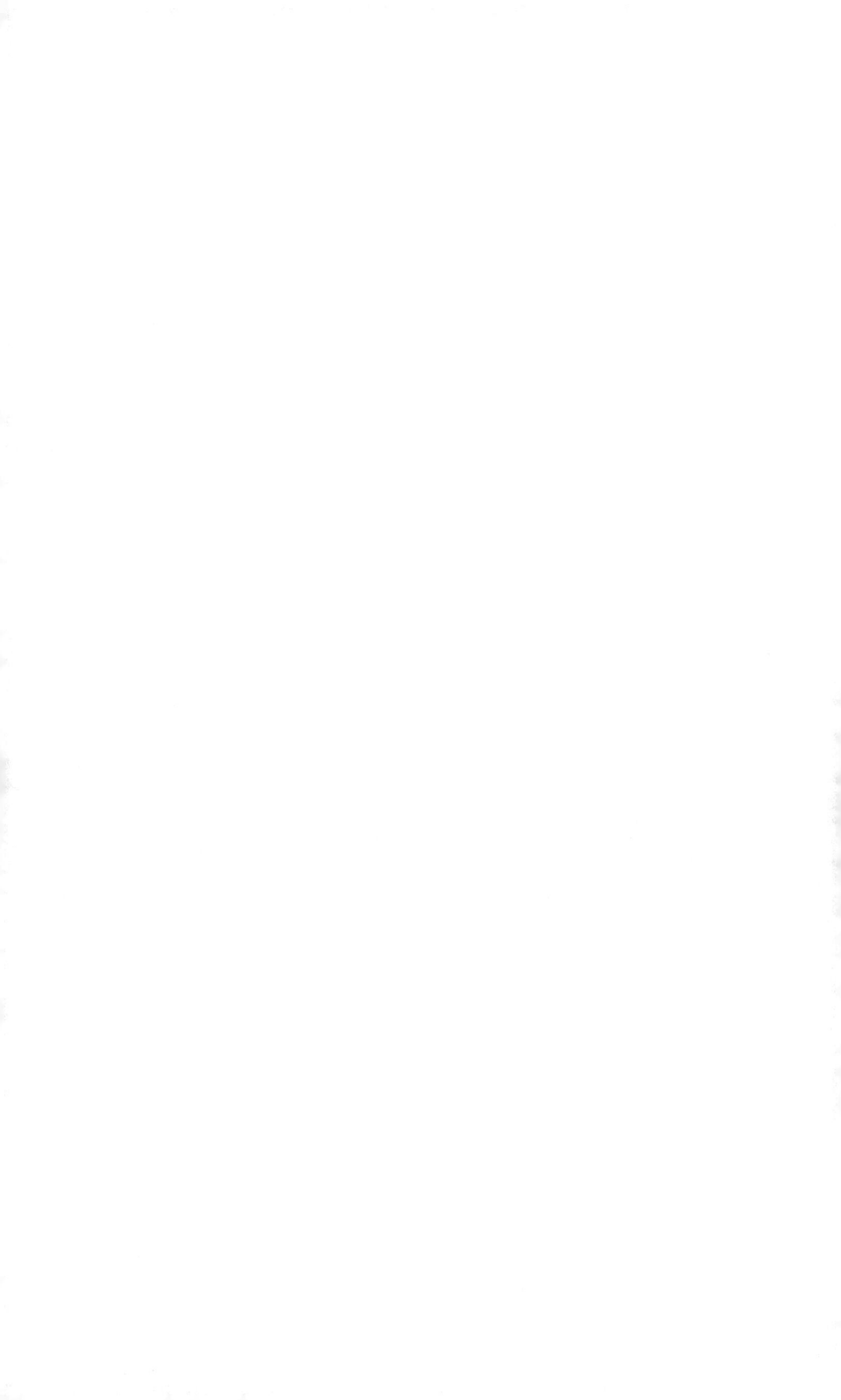